Distribution, publication, and copying in any form are prohibited and subject to damages.

TEN HYPNOSES

Copying, publishing, and sharing with third parties are only permitted with the written consent of the author. Please observe the notes on copyright and usage.

Distribution, publication, and copying in any form are prohibited and subject to damages.

Copying, publishing, and sharing with third parties are only permitted with the written consent of the author. Please observe the notes on copyright and usage.

Ingo Michael Simon

TEN HYPNOSES

34
ANTICIPATORY ANXIETY, FEAR OF FEAR

Distribution, publication, and copying in any form are prohibited and subject to damages.

© 2024 Ingo Michael Simon
All rights reserved.
Independently published
www.ingosimon.com

Important Notes for Urgent Attention:

The contents of this book are based on the practical experiences of the author with hypnosis applications and psychotherapy in a trance state. Although the author has strived for the utmost care, errors or misunderstandings in the presentation cannot be completely excluded. Therapeutic work with people and the application of hypnosis are solely the responsibility of the hypnotist. It cannot be ruled out that parts of this book may be misunderstood or that the application of a presented procedure may cause an undesirable reaction in the client. The author also assumes no co-responsibility if work with a client is carried out with reference to the statements in this book.

The Author:

Ingo Michael Simon studied psychology and education and is a hypnotherapist with practices in southwestern Germany and Switzerland. With the help of hypnosis-supported psychotherapy, he primarily treats people with persistent psychological conditions. His practice focuses on anxiety disorders, pathological compulsions, and psychosomatic illnesses. His therapeutic offerings mainly include classical and modern hypnosis applications and the dreamland therapy he developed himself.

Copying, publishing, and sharing with third parties are only permitted with the written consent of the author. Please observe the notes on copyright and usage.

Distribution, publication, and copying in any form are prohibited and subject to damages.

INTRODUCTION	**6**
COPYRIGHT AND USAGE	**8**
HYPNOSIS 1	**10**
HYPNOSIS 2	**15**
HYPNOSIS 3	**20**
HYPNOSIS 4	**26**
HYPNOSIS 5	**30**
HYPNOSIS 6	**35**
HYPNOSIS 7	**40**
HYPNOSIS 8	**45**
HYPNOSIS 9	**51**
HYPNOSIS 10	**56**
ALL TITLES IN THE SERIES	**61**

Copying, publishing, and sharing with third parties are only permitted with the written consent of the author. Please observe the notes on copyright and usage.

Distribution, publication, and copying in any form are prohibited and subject to damages.

Introduction

The series "Ten Hypnoses" is very well known in Germany, Austria, and Switzerland as a collection of texts for therapeutic work and is used by numerous psychotherapeutic practices, doctors, therapists, coaches, and other helping professionals. I am pleased to now be able to offer these texts in other countries as well.

Most therapists have their own methods for inducing and deepening trance as well as for exiting trance. Therefore, I have focused on the main part of the hypnosis. The texts in this book can be integrated as the main part into any hypnosis process. The texts in this collection use various hypnosis techniques. I will not explain these in detail, as I assume that users have the appropriate training. It is also not necessary to understand the exact structure or functioning of the different parts. The texts can simply be read aloud, and they will have their effect.

Decide for yourself which text best suits your client or patient at any given time. You can also combine passages from different texts. It is not about using all ten hypnoses in sequence. It is a selection of possibilities.

Copying, publishing, and sharing with third parties are only permitted with the written consent of the author. Please observe the notes on copyright and usage.

I want to emphasize that books cannot replace therapy. Psychotherapy or other therapeutic treatments involve much more. A careful diagnosis is the necessary basis for deciding on the use of methods, including whether hypnosis or one of my texts should be used. Even in this case, preparatory discussions, follow-up discussions during the session, and of course, a therapeutic concept for the sequence of sessions and the content approaches are essential parts of therapy. This cannot and should not be achieved with a collection of texts.

In any case, I wish you much success in your work and I am pleased if my text templates can contribute in a small way.

Ingo Michael Simon

Distribution, publication, and copying in any form are prohibited and subject to damages.

Copyright and Usage

Copying, publishing, and sharing with third parties is prohibited and only permitted with the written consent of the author. Please observe the following copyright and usage guidelines.

This work has been carefully crafted and created to the best of the author's knowledge and personal experience. It comprises text templates and application guidelines for professional hypnosis sessions. The author is a licensed psychotherapist with extensive experience in psychotherapy, coaching, and personal training using hypnotic techniques and methods. Nevertheless, the author and the publisher assume no liability for the accuracy of information, instructions, and advice, nor for any typographical errors. The author and publisher accept no responsibility or liability for the application of these texts and recommendations with clients or patients, nor for any potential consequences or unexpected reactions. It is expressly noted that the application of therapeutic and advisory techniques and formulations lies solely and entirely within the responsibility of the practitioner. This also applies to adherence to the

Copying, publishing, and sharing with third parties are only permitted with the written consent of the author. Please observe the notes on copyright and usage.

boundaries of legally regulated medical and therapeutic practices. The fact that a book containing action proposals is freely available for sale does not imply that its application with clients or patients is permitted for everyone.

Hypnosis 1

You've decided that today is the day to end those fearful thoughts... to put an end to the anticipation of fear... You want to be free again and feel good... You want to replace those thoughts of fear... You want to replace the expectation of fear with a new inner freedom... This is possible, and that's why you're here today... because you can do it... You can and you will do it... You've set your mind to this... and that's the right step because it's truly our thoughts that can influence and control our feelings... So, you're fully focusing on the single thought of ending the anticipation of fear... today... right now... It's remarkable how quickly you can embrace this thought as the most important one... because nothing is more important right now than freeing yourself from those fearful thoughts... Today, you're following this thought of liberation...

You've had many stressful thoughts of fear... Often, it's been the anticipation of a fear attack that has actually produced fear, even when no attack occurred... Your thoughts raced ahead of the actual fear... even before a fear attack could manifest... Today, you realize that it was this anticipation that caused most of the restlessness and fear... this fear that rushed ahead and allowed nothing else but fear... But today, your thoughts are changing, and this is possible because you now understand and fully embrace the idea that focused thoughts can control your feelings... So, we can also turn the thought around, and you can consciously choose to think a thought of calm or security, ensuring that you truly have calm thoughts and feel safe... That's what you need... security... So, let this new thought grow... It says... I am doing well, and I am happy about it... It's a simple thought, but because of that, it's a very good thought—one that does more than that... It's a thought that ensures your feelings remain good... without fear... with confidence and calmness... with joy and with peace...

Your body also aligns with your thoughts... The anticipation of fear could create tension in your body... perhaps cause muscle tension or stomach aches... Relaxed thoughts, on the other hand, can have a relaxing and calming effect on your body... So, consciously feel your body now... It is relaxed... It is truly relaxed right now... This is only possible because there are already calm and relaxed thoughts within you… This shows you that calm and constructive, helpful thoughts are already within you, helping you… That's the only way your body can be relaxed now… because you're not waiting for fear right now… because right now, you're only expecting calmness and relaxation… Your body is relaxed, even though—or maybe precisely because—I'm talking about fear the entire time… Your body doesn't react with fear at all because there are thoughts of freedom within you… perhaps in your subconscious, but they are there… Your body shows you with its relaxation that you have already let go of the fearful thoughts and are becoming free… I say fear, and you remain relaxed… You've let go of the anticipation of fear… Isn't that wonderful? … You've already freed yourself…

Now enjoy the feeling of inner relaxation… Focus your awareness on the feeling of relaxation within you… Feel the calmness and peace… Also, feel the pleasant drowsiness inviting you to do nothing… just to be here, because that's enough… Right now, in your calm feeling, just being here is enough… Turn your gaze inward and feel deep inside… There you find a beautiful and pleasant calmness… There you find an inviting drowsiness and true freedom… Let these feelings be present now... Let them spread... Allow your pleasant feelings to spread completely now... The more you can now feel a pleasant feeling, the freer you will become... because pleasant feelings and the anticipation of fear can never exist simultaneously... So, focus now on a pleasant feeling and let go of the anticipation of fear... Focus on a pleasant feeling and become free... Now...

Now, at this very moment, it becomes normal for you to focus primarily on a pleasant feeling... and with that, you feel good... You know that there are always multiple feelings present at the same time... There are always many feelings within us... so it's about directing your attention and awareness to a feeling that makes the anticipation of fear impossible... a feeling that sets you free... Every pleasant feeling drives away fear and sets you free... Every pleasant feeling you can perceive helps you to let go of fear... now and every day... You can always and at any time find the feeling of hope when you focus on your inner self... You can always and at any time find the feeling of confidence when you focus on your inner self... And whenever you focus on a feeling and turn toward it, it immediately becomes significant and helps you... A little hope becomes big when you focus on it... Some calmness becomes deep calmness when you focus on it... Now... Awareness and concentration strengthen pleasant feelings... and with that, you let go of the anticipation of fear and become free... free again and again...

You've changed your inner perspective... Today, you've turned toward yourself, and with that, you can always ensure that pleasant feelings spread and fear fades away... You can ensure every day that you think and feel... I am doing well, and I am happy about it... because it's your attention that guides your thoughts and your feelings... because you decide with your inner gaze which thoughts and which feelings become clear... And you choose beautiful and pleasant feelings, today and every day...

Hypnosis 2

You've decided to let go of those fearful thoughts today... You want to and you will let go of the anticipation of fear today... You know the feeling of waiting for fear, and you've experienced that it often doesn't come... that's why today it's also possible to end this expectation... You're focusing on your goal to remain calm again and to clearly feel self-confidence and self-assurance... Today, you really succeed in distancing yourself from and even letting go of the anticipation of fear... Today, you even manage to look forward to the new and unexpected... You can do this because you are safe... Today, you are completely reorienting yourself deep inside... Your thoughts are once again following your will, and you want to be free... Your thoughts are once again following your will, and you want to let go of fear... Your thoughts are once again following your will, and you want to be self-assured... Your thoughts are once again following your will, and you want to feel true, genuine self-confidence... because with that, the anticipation of fear becomes impossible... You're expecting good feelings and experiences...

Remember a success now, whatever comes to mind... There have been successes in your life... big and seemingly small ones, which always felt big at the moment of success... With the thought of success, you feel a sensation... It's a feeling of inner strength and power... You can feel it because it's there... Often, your own inner strength has helped you to get through challenging situations; you've even endured situations of fear and kept going... So, you can do it today too... You are strong, and your strength is now becoming clearer and clearer... It's increasingly coming into your awareness... You are truly strong, and you're awakening this great strength within you today... because your own strength helps you to let go of the anticipation of fear... Today, you are stronger than ever before, much stronger than ever before... and you can use this special power today to truly let go of those fearful thoughts... You really have the power...

You're reorienting yourself deep within to new thoughts... Today, you're finding thoughts of relaxation... thoughts of calm... But before that, it's about letting go of those fearful thoughts... letting go of the anticipation of fear... Today, you let go of the anticipation and the fearful thoughts... You succeed today in experiencing inner relaxation again... Now you truly let go of fear deep within and, with that, also in your thoughts... With this, you're already reorienting yourself toward calmness and serenity... You're experiencing inner freedom again... Today is the day when everything changes... because today you are truly freeing yourself from fearful thoughts, and you're becoming inwardly calm... You can feel it within you... You can feel it more and more clearly... You are relaxed and calm...

With this inner release of fear, a free space is created... A free space that you can use... A free space for new and very pleasant thoughts that are allowed to spread on their own... The thought of a new expectation arises within you... Where the anticipation of fear once was, there is now free space, and the expectation of the beautiful new is emerging... You look forward to the new things in your life... Each day brings you new and unexpectedly beautiful experiences... Today and with each passing day, you succeed in truly looking forward to the new... You succeed in embracing life with joy again... lightheartedly and full of confidence... Trusting thoughts are growing stronger and spreading... Now, true trust is really emerging again... fundamental trust in life and in yourself... You trust life... You trust yourself above all, because you are becoming freer and freer...

You have already overcome many challenges in your life and have repeatedly freed yourself from difficult situations... Today, too, you've overcome a difficult situation and taken a step towards freedom... You've succeeded today in letting go of the anticipation of fear... Truly remarkable how quickly you've been able to reorient yourself and have already let go of the anticipation of fear... Truly very impressive and very composed because you've actually done it... You've let go of the fear of fear... You've refocused on your confidence... on your self-confidence... Today, you've truly undergone an inner transformation... You've undergone a significant inner transformation today... You've first transformed the anticipation of fear into calmness and then into self-confidence... Self-confidence that helps you to look forward to the new again... to turn to life again with curiosity and interest... free and calm... You can do it... You are free... You can really do it... You are truly free... You can do more today than you thought... You've really and finally freed yourself, and you've succeeded in letting go of those fearful thoughts... Now...

Today, you've created real freedom for yourself... This new and genuine freedom remains... because everything you achieve here in trance, every step you take in trance... becomes a reality in your waking life... Freedom and self-confidence remain with you in your waking life... Freedom and calmness... Self-confidence and inner strength remain with you in your waking life, truly... You are free today and tomorrow... and every day of your life to come, you can experience freedom and self-confidence anew... From now on, everything is different... because from now on, you feel more self-confidence and more self-assurance than before... You know that you have relaxed thoughts... You know that you await everything new and unexpected with calm interest...

Hypnosis 3

Guidelines for Use:

In this hypnosis session, a post-hypnotic anchor is used. An anchor (or trigger) is a stimulus that is meant to evoke a specific feeling or thought. It acts as a signal that the client perceives, which then triggers an internal process. The anchor replaces the suggestion, and the client can use it in everyday life to trigger a desired state, even outside of trance. Many stimuli can be used as anchors/triggers. In my practice, I use the following options, also found in the series "Ten Hypnoses":

- **Physical Anchors:** Closing the hand, pressing the ball of the thumb, etc.
- **Visual Anchors:** Symbols, word cards, etc.
- **Auditory Anchors:** Sound signals like phone rings, melodies, etc.
- **Olfactory Anchors:** Scented oils, etc.
- **Tactile Anchors:** Smooth stones, talismans, etc.

Additionally, I distinguish between perihypnotic and posthypnotic anchors. Perihypnotic anchors are used primarily during hypnosis, where the therapist sets up the anchor and then triggers it repeatedly as an enhancement to suggestions and visualizations. Posthypnotic anchors are primarily set up for use after the session, allowing the client to help themselves with the anchor.

+++ End of Guidelines +++

Today, we're going to establish an anchor together… This is a small but very effective tool designed to help you let go of the anticipation of fear and then remain truly free from it… Like an anchor that keeps a ship safe in place even during a storm, your anchor will help you stay in a place of control, always maintaining control over the situation… especially when a feeling of fear or anticipation of fear might arise… Then your anchor will provide you with control and bring you back to a calm state, where you'll remain… You can carry your anchor with you, as it's portable… Initially, it will help you stay calm or become calmer when fear might arise… and eventually, it will act as an anchor, constantly ensuring that fear can't arise, as you'll be able to use it immediately if even the slightest fearful thought arises...

[Hold a small softball that can be easily squeezed. It should be only two or three centimeters in diameter so that it can be carried around easily in everyday life. When you later give the ball to the client, announce briefly that you are going to hand them the ball and then touch the client's hand with the softball so that they can grasp it. Simply follow the cues in the text! Suitable balls can be found in pet stores as toys for very small dogs.]

But first, you need to be truly free of fear... right now, truly free of fear in this very moment... But that's really easy, because right now, you're completely relaxed and have no anticipation of fear, not now... You feel good, and you are calm... after all, you're in a comfortable trance and therefore also relaxed... In relaxation, fear cannot exist... Only one can exist—relaxation or fear... And right now, it's definitely relaxation... only relaxation... Now the relaxation goes even deeper... and in this state of relaxation, you also feel completely free from fear... You're now waiting for even more relaxation... You're now waiting for even deeper relaxation... The more you focus on the feeling of relaxation now, in this moment... in this very moment... the better you can actually feel that fear is not present at all... You don't have to worry about anything now... You don't have to achieve anything now... Now, you have peace... You are relaxed... You are tired... You are completely calm...

Now, in this deep relaxation, you can also simply let go of all possible anticipations of fear and feel free... It's no longer even possible to wait for fear now... Now, you can only think and feel calmness... You are now truly calm, relaxed, and free from fear... The more clearly you can feel the relaxation now, the better you can feel free... So, feel the relaxation and accept yourself and this beautiful calmness... Now... Now it's happening... Feel the relaxation now and accept yourself and this deep calmness... Now it's happening... Now I'm giving you the relaxation ball in your hand... [Touch the client's hand and give them the softball. They can keep their eyes closed.]... Feel the relaxation ball in your hand... Feel the relaxation and squeeze the ball now... Feel the relaxation... good... once more... Feel the calmness within you and enjoy the calm feeling and squeeze the ball... Excellent... It works... Your body understands... Your deep inner self has understood and learned for you... Squeeze the ball once more... good... This is your relaxation ball... This is your "fear-away" ball... The ball really helps you, because whenever you squeeze it, just like now, you feel so relaxed and calm... Whenever you squeeze the ball, just like now, any possible fear disappears... Whenever you squeeze the ball, just like now, you become calm and stay calm... With your "fear-away" ball, you quickly become calm inside... just like now... exactly like now... When you squeeze the ball, your entire body, your entire organism remembers the relaxation and stays relaxed... Your anchor helps you with this... You know that you can free yourself from fear again and again... just like today... The softball helps you with that... This ball in your hands is your anchor... the anchor that holds you firmly in calmness... the anchor that prevents you from slipping into fear... You don't go into fear; you stay in safety... you stay in this safe feeling that you're feeling right now, because your anchor brings you there and keeps you there... Your anchor brings you into a calm feeling and keeps you in that calm feeling...

You can carry the ball with you every day... and whenever you feel like fearful thoughts are following you, just squeeze it... and fear disappears... and you become calm... With each squeeze of the ball, you become calmer every day... The ball helps you every day... You did it... You've really already done it... You've freed yourself... and every day, you free yourself again if you want... with your "fear-away" ball...

Hypnosis 4

Today, you want to let go of fearful thoughts; that's your goal... The time of anticipating fear should come to an end, to be replaced by a new time of good feelings and pleasant expectations... You've had this goal for a long time, but today, it's within reach... Today, you want to end the anticipation of fear... and more than that... You want to be able to look forward to what's coming, to be open to the events and experiences of the day... because you want to feel free, truly free... You want to feel free because you are free... You want to feel free... because as soon as you've succeeded in turning your goal into a deep inner conviction, you'll feel truly free... truly free... and filled with new, good thoughts and feelings... This is possible... this is truly possible today, and you can do it... Today, you free yourself once and for all...

Let's begin... First, it's about letting go of disturbing thoughts, and that's easy when you focus on a specific image... Just imagine sitting in a cone of light... A cone of radiant, golden light, and you're sitting comfortably in the middle, in complete serenity... Your gaze gets lost in the golden light that surrounds you, that's around you and envelops you... You see and feel the golden light around you and find a pleasant calmness deep within you... All thoughts fade away... It's as if all your thoughts are being dissolved by the golden light, and you come to rest... You now allow yourself deep rest... You see and feel only the golden light that flows through your skin into your body and makes you calmer and calmer... Golden light flows through your body and makes you calm...

Then your gaze goes deeper and deeper into the light... It's as if you could look through the golden light and see into infinity... And before your inner eye, a script appears with words that you can understand and accept as your affirmation, as your inner belief... You recognize this script in the golden light... It stands there, in the infinity of space, written in clear letters just for you... It says...

I open myself to all my good and pleasant feelings, and I look forward to peace and calm.

... [Read the affirmation slowly and slightly louder than the previous text to highlight it a bit. Then pause for about 30 seconds before continuing.]

And now allow this affirmation to unfold its effect within you... because that's exactly what's happening now, as this affirmation aligns with your desires and goals... And it truly does, because you want to rediscover and use the good feelings of peace and calm for yourself... You want to be relaxed again and experience calm thoughts... Your affirmation, this inner belief, becomes the new truth in your life as soon as it aligns with your goals... and it already does... So now it's time to experience this new truth... This special phrase now becomes a new and deep belief within you...

This new belief becomes your deep conviction today... a conviction that you can repeat and use like an inner creed... like a mantra from you for yourself...

I open myself to all my good and pleasant feelings, and I look forward to peace and calm.

... Now take a deep breath in and out... Let your breath flow consciously into your lungs... Feel the path of your breath in your body... Feel how you take in this fresh air and how it fills your body... and with this deep breath, you also take in your affirmation... With every further deep breath, it's as if you're breathing in your affirmation, your belief, and letting it flow deep into your innermost being... Good... That's right...

That's really good, you did it... You've really done it... You've truly embraced this new attitude of inner freedom because now you feel calm, relaxed, and free... In your waking life, you will feel this effect... You will feel in your waking life that you truly have relaxed thoughts... You won't expect fear at all anymore... and if you want to strengthen the effect so that fearful thoughts can't arise at all, then just consciously and intentionally say to yourself... I open myself to all my good and pleasant feelings, and I look forward to peace and calm... and immediately your entire organism goes into a calm state that you can clearly feel... You've done it... You've succeeded, and with that, you succeed every day anew... You start each new day with a moment of calmness, and then you say your affirmation once and start your day lightly...

Hypnosis 5

You've made a decision... The fear of future fears should go away... You want to end these worries... You want to free yourself... because that's what you really need... freedom... and that's exactly what's possible today... Today, more than ever... Today, you can achieve more than ever... because you've decided... because you're here and consciously walking this path... You're succeeding... It's truly amazing how much you've already set yourself up to let go of fear and feel free again from today on... I'm here to help you with this very liberation...

Imagine that your fears are like small beads of thought in your head... like little beads that are in your head and move around among all your other thoughts... and each fear has its own color... Breathe in and out and imagine that your breath flows through your entire head... If you can imagine that, then you can also imagine that your thoughts are being swirled around by the air flowing into your head... and some of them can even be exhaled... Perhaps it can't be any other way, because with every exhale, the air flows out of your head and always takes some thought beads with it... You can imagine it; it's quite easy... and if you can imagine that, then you can also imagine that you can gather certain thoughts and then exhale them... So, begin... Find the fearful thoughts and breathe them out... I'm here to help you... There are different types of fears... There are the unpredictable fears that come suddenly and unexpectedly... that have surprised you... They carry the color red... All the red thought beads represent sudden fears... Then there are also predictable fears, perhaps situations that have often made you afraid and that you can foresee well... They move around as brown thought beads in your head... And finally, there's the fear of fear itself, the anxious expectation of the next fear attack... You know this fear... It has been there very often... This fear of fear, which we also call anticipatory anxiety, is yellow... In your head, you can find lots of yellow fearful thoughts... lots of yellow thought beads... Today, you can let go of all these thoughts... Today, you can get rid of all these disturbing fearful thoughts and become free...

Now, imagine how it often was when the fears came... It was as if certain thoughts suddenly became very big, very prominent... Suddenly, all the brown thoughts were there and occupied your attention... But actually, all the other thoughts were always there too, especially thoughts and feelings that had nothing to do with fear... beautiful thoughts... strong thoughts... and thoughts of calmness and self-control... All these good and helpful thoughts are green... And there really are plenty of green thoughts in your head... Today, you can ensure that the fearful thoughts go away, and then mainly good green thoughts remain... This is possible because you are here... because you are in trance and can achieve much more in trance than in your waking life...

Imagine that your breath is magnetic and can gather the thoughts of your choice... Simply start with the red thoughts... Breathe in deeply and gather all the red thoughts... and with the next breath, breathe out the red thought beads... They tumble out of your nose and turn into bubbles that float through the room... As soon as the red thought beads of sudden fear leave your nose, they expand like soap bubbles and float through the room and burst... And with that, you become freer and lighter... and find more and more good green thoughts that remain within you... Stand beside yourself and watch as the red thought beads of sudden fear leave your nose and float as bubbles through the room... And one after another, they burst... Fear dissolves, and you become light inside... Then you also breathe out the brown thought beads, and they too expand and float as brown bubbles through the room... bubbles of predictable fears... You breathe them all out... And the brown bubbles of fear burst... Fear dissolves, and you become light inside... You discover more and more good green thoughts that remain within you; they are pleasant and helpful... [Fifteen seconds of silence]... And now the yellow thoughts of anticipatory anxiety... The yellow thought beads of waiting for the next fear attack... You breathe them out... They tumble out of your nose as yellow beads, and you can see them, watch them... And then they expand and float as delicate bubbles through the room... And one fear after another bursts... All the fears burst... Fear dissolves, and you become light inside... The red thought beads disappear... The brown thought beads disappear... The yellow thought beads disappear... Beautiful green thoughts spread... Beautiful green thoughts spread...

Your deep inner self is now completely adjusting to breathing out fearful thoughts every day and letting them burst as bubbles... because breathing out the fearful thoughts helps you become free again and again... to find new beautiful thoughts and feel free... You perceive your feelings, and you accept them, and if they are fearful feelings, then you breathe them out as thought beads again and again... You feel free... You truly feel free... now and every day...

Hypnosis 6

This is the goal today: ending the anticipation of fear... This fear has truly served its time and should end today... It's an expectation... an expectation of fear, but the waiting is over... The fear is over... today... now... Fear should go away today so that you can finally feel free again, truly free... The memory of fear becomes harmless today because the fear is over... The idea of experiencing another fear attack becomes harmless because you know that you are much stronger than fear... Thoughts of fear should be indifferent and remain indifferent... That's your goal... That's today's goal... the most important goal, and this goal is the focus of your trance today... the focus of your will... Today, you're already freeing yourself from all anticipations of fear... Today, you're already freeing yourself from fear... today... now...

Deep within you, in your subconscious, there is a very special place... It's a place where special encounters can take place when you're in trance... Today, an encounter can happen there that really helps you to let go of those fearful thoughts... to let go of the anticipation of fear... It's an encounter with yourself... We could also say with a part of you... with a powerful part of you... This place within you is a place of freedom and opportunities... a place of limitless possibilities... You find it beyond your waking mind... This is only possible in trance, and now you are in trance... here and now... because you are in this deep state of relaxation, where you can turn your gaze inward and see everything that belongs to you... Turn your gaze inward now... similar to falling asleep and gradually starting to dream... You dream yourself to this special place within you... A special encounter is waiting for you there...

There is someone with you, and you have the feeling that this person is very much like you... It's an encounter in feeling, familiar and unique... You feel safe and secure because this special place is the safest place in the world... It lies within you, and deep inside you are truly safe... Then you feel your hand being touched, and it feels like a very familiar hand is reaching for yours... and slowly an inner image forms at the place of the encounter, and you can recognize the person who has taken your hand to help you... It's yourself, standing there like a twin brother/sister [Please adjust to the client's gender] facing you... Your mirror image holds your hand to show you that you are not alone... that you always have a partner by your side... You are that partner yourself... A very strong and powerful part of you is that partner...

This part of you knows your fear and your anticipation of fear... This helper within you is here to help you now... to help you let go of the anticipation of fear... and to feel free again... This part of you understands you... You've often lacked understanding... You've experienced that others couldn't understand that you were afraid of fear itself... You thought you were crazy... But you are perfectly normal... You've had fearful thoughts, but you are normal... and your helper knows this and also knows the causes and connections of fear and anticipation of fear... But knowing the reasons and origins isn't always so important; what's most important is finding a way out of those fearful thoughts... And your helper is here today to show you that there is a way... to show you that way today and help you walk it today... Deep inside, you feel connected and safe... connected with yourself and completely safe... and with every breath, you feel a little freer... because your fearful thoughts are being taken up by your helper... Every memory of fear, every fear you once had, and every memory of the anxious anticipation of the next fear... All of this flows from within you through your hand to the hand of your helper, who gladly takes this fear from you... Your helper is a part of you... and so your anticipation of fear flows from your thoughts to this special part of you... to the part of you that can truly process this fear deep inside... so deep inside that the fear is no longer in your thoughts and you become free... Your helper can now start to dissolve this fear deep inside, calmly and slowly processing and dissolving the causes and connections deep in your subconscious... This really works... because now you're meeting yourself on this special level... You, in your waking life, can now feel comfortable again and enjoy light thoughts... You hand over your anticipation of fear to yourself, but you hand it over to a part of you that can handle it well and successfully deep inside... Your helper is this inner part that takes the fear with it and can process and dissolve it deep inside... This really works, and it will succeed if you hand over all fearful thoughts... They are now flowing from your hand to the helping hand...

Let it all happen and allow this inner part to do the work for you... Your subconscious is happy to help you and gladly does this work for you... Everything now happens on its own... Your anticipation of fear flows more and more inward, so your thoughts become free again... That's right, your inner helper is doing this for you... and you're slowly returning to the outside... from hand to hand, you remain connected to your inner helper and return to the outside...

Hypnosis 7

You want to end the anticipation of fear today... You want to experience your everyday life calmly and let it come to you... There was a time when you didn't even think about something like anticipating fear or the next fear attack... because it simply didn't exist... You didn't have panic attacks; they only developed later... So, you didn't have any fear of the next attack back then... You don't need to know the reasons for all these fears... To free yourself from them, you only need to go on a special journey... now...

The journey begins... your journey through the course of your life... through images and impressions that are in your memory... through the feelings and moods you once had... Nothing is ever lost; everything experienced remains as a memory in our feelings, and we can find it all again... Perhaps there are many experiences you can remember well... Perhaps it's like a movie you can watch, running backward... Or your journey is like wandering through colors and shapes... Maybe it's sounds accompanying you on your journey... melodies of everyday life... Or maybe there's a bit of everything, and lively memories come alive... There was a time before anticipatory anxiety... a time when you let life's events come to you... without worry... without fear... without expecting fear... On your journey today, you are getting closer and closer to this time... Your journey today goes back to a time before the anticipation of fear and even further... to a time before fear altogether... Back then, you hadn't experienced any panic attacks... Back then, you only knew ordinary fear in dangerous situations... It's as if you're jumping back into a time without fear... For this, you don't have to do anything special or come up with a trick... You don't have to remember something very specific or think of a particular event... Just imagine that you arrive at a time before fear on your inner journey... Now... There are no panic attacks and no anticipation of fear, and there never were...

Now feel yourself into that earlier time... Feel your emotions... Feel once more the sense of life of that time... the freedom from fear and, with it, the calmness and peace... That was completely natural for you back then... calmness and peace... That was truly natural, and you remember it... Feel inside yourself... Sense what time you are in... in what time of your life... Feel your age... perhaps you are much younger or even a child... Sense the feeling you had at that time and that you still have... because all feelings remain... They are still there and can help you... Look around, see where you are, where your journey has led you... and then let these images be there and become clearer... The time before the fear becomes clearer and clearer... You are back in your thoughts to the truly fearless time... You are in a calm feeling... And the good and strong feelings from back then are awakened... It's your old calmness that you can feel again... Your old calmness is reactivated... You feel this calmness, which becomes clearer and clearer... your calmness... It's your calmness because you had it back then and still have it today... Calmness from you, for you... There are other strengths within you that you are rediscovering... Another strong and helpful feeling is now awakening within you... a feeling that was natural back then and is again completely natural today and helps you... A feeling or an ability that helps you to let go of anticipatory anxiety once and for all... Your strengths are becoming active and are imprinting themselves firmly on you so that you can use them at any time and again and again to free yourself from fearful thoughts…

Today, you're reclaiming your own abilities and holding them tight… they are your abilities… So, you can also hold onto them… feel them and anchor them firmly within you… You feel these constructive feelings in your body; you can even take them with you… Filled with your own strengths, free from fear and with positive expectations, your journey now continues… Your journey now takes you into the future… You go into a near future to recognize that you are truly succeeding in taking your strengths with you and remaining free… You're taking a journey into the future… From the fearless past, you now take a big inner step into an equally fearless future… into a future where you also don't anticipate fear because you've already left it behind… In the future, you only expect your own strengths… You are now on your inner journey into a fearless future… maybe a few months ahead or only a few weeks or just days… and there you stop, in a fearless near future… You no longer have panic attacks in this fearless future… You no longer have anticipatory anxiety in this near future; it's simply no longer possible… You look at how it is to experience your everyday life calmly... You can already feel inside you how easy it has become to really experience and actively shape your everyday life with calmness and serenity... You can do it... You can do it today... You can do it... Yes, you can...

Good... Now you can calmly return to the present... to now also enjoy your everyday life in the present, in your waking life... free from expectations... free from fear... with calmness... with self-confidence... with inner peace... You succeed... You've already succeeded... because everything you can feel on an inner journey, you can also feel in waking life, just a few moments later... and in a few moments, you'll be awake again... and then the new time has already become the present...

Hypnosis 8

Guidelines for Use:

This hypnosis session uses ideomotor signaling. Ideomotor signaling refers to the phenomenon where our body responds to our feelings and thoughts with movements. In everyday life, this response is seen in posture, muscle tension, and movement patterns that naturally change with one's mood and thoughts. In trance, ideomotor signals can be used to obtain information that the client cannot actively communicate. The subconscious can, for example, respond to questions with an agreed-upon finger signal. Of course, ideomotor reactions can also be used suggestively, such as in arm levitation and catalepsy. An ideomotor approach strengthens trust in hypnosis and one's ability to change, thus promoting therapy.

+++ End of Guidelines +++

Today, you want to dissolve the fear of fear... This is possible because a special part of you can do it... This special part of you can actually be reached and commissioned in trance... Many things are possible in trance because, in trance, you can directly address your subconscious and commission it to let go of fear for you... Perhaps you're already aware that your fear is a signal from your subconscious... But it's not really about fear... Fear is an invitation from your subconscious to come closer and connect with it... Then fear can go away... This special part of you, the unconscious or subconscious, no longer needs fear... for that, I need to speak directly with your subconscious... You, stay in a beautiful fantasy... Imagine the most beautiful fantasy you can think of... and stay in this beautiful idea... You can understand every word you hear from me, but just stay in your beautiful fantasy and imagine that all thoughts, ideas, and fantasies are going to the left... into the left side of your body... and you, the subconscious of [Client's First Name], come to the right and move into the right hand... and give me a signal with a finger of the right hand as soon as you've managed to reach the hand... While the waking mind remains in a beautiful fantasy on the left, you, the subconscious of [Client's First Name], come to the right and move a finger of the right hand...

... [Be patient and stay with it. Don't worry—finger signals (almost) always work! Repeat the prompt several times kindly and with some insistence, and exude confidence. If you're sure that a finger signal will come, it will happen faster than if you doubt it.]

... ... There's the signal, good... Thank you... Now, subconscious of [Client's First Name], make sure the waking mind is dreaming deeply on the left side so that we can work well together... The greeting finger shall be the yes-finger... For each confirmation, you can move it... For rejection, you can move another finger... Choose a finger for no now and move it... [Wait for the finger signal!] ... Thank you... We now have the [Yes-Finger] for yes and the [No-Finger] for no... So, we can begin... We can now start dissolving the fear for good...

... Are you ready? ... [Wait for Yes-Finger!] ... Good, let's go...

Subconscious of [Client's First Name], we understand that anticipation of fear has causes, but we don't know exactly what they are... I know that you're trying to build a better communication with the waking mind, with reason. I also know that the fear disappears when your messages and communications are received differently. I want to help you find a new path without fearful thoughts, and the waking mind will make an effort in everyday life to stay in touch with you with mindfulness... But you have to do it, because you, subconscious of [Client's First Name], can do it... For yes, please use the yes-finger, and for no, the agreed-upon no-finger... Let's start...

... Now, find a way to communicate with the waking mind from the endless variety of possibilities within you. This path must have nothing to do with fear. It must be pleasant so that it can truly succeed... Show me with the yes-finger once you've found a good way... [Wait for Yes-Finger!] ... Good, you've found a new way... But we want to be sure that this also works well... Imagine how it is in your everyday life... in a situation where fearful thoughts often came... Imagine now that you're choosing another inner path there, a path only you know, one that you've now chosen... a new path of communication with the waking mind... Test whether this path works without fear and give me a signal...

... if yes ... Excellent, your new path works and it works without fearful thoughts...

... if no ... It's not yet the best path... Find another good path of communication and show me with the yes-finger once you've found another path without fear... [Wait for Yes-Finger and repeat as many times as necessary until it's shown! Don't worry, this happens after at most three tries!]... Excellent, your new path works without fearful thoughts...

... Subconscious of [Client's Name], you see that we are making an effort together to understand and help you... The waking mind and I... And we will continue to do so, and I promise you that the waking mind will continue to make an effort to understand your messages and communications... That's what the waking mind does for you... What you must do is use your new path without fearful thoughts. Only if there's no other way, you briefly use the fearful thoughts... Agreed?... [A no will not come here] ... Then, now set everything up inside you so that you use this path instead of the fearful thoughts from now on... Whenever and whatever you, subconscious of [Client's First Name], want to communicate to your own waking mind, your reason, from now on, you use your new path, without fear... Show me with the yes-finger when you're finished with that... Show me with the yes-finger that you've firmly established this new path... [Wait for Yes-Finger]

Good, it's done... You, subconscious of [Client's First Name], can thoroughly test your new time without anticipations of fear until we meet again... and if your new path works so well, you can then keep it forever or even expand and optimize it...

Hypnosis 9

Guidelines for Use:

In this hypnosis session, a self-hypnosis trigger is established. A self-hypnosis trigger is a signal that initiates the state of trance. With its help, even an inexperienced client can continue working with self-hypnosis at home. Of course, they can "only" work with simple suggestions that they can easily remember and that we should prepare, or with simple visualizations. Triggered self-hypnosis is a very good tool to give the client a task to continue the therapy. This way, the time between sessions in the practice isn't without therapy but is continued at home. Fully self-directed self-hypnosis, without a trigger, is also well-learned but requires much time and practice. Setting up the trigger is a fairly simple task and, of course, relieves the client, who I don't want to burden with the training of self-directed self-hypnosis. Despite all the naysayers, I also claim here that it's really not a problem to teach a client simple trigger self-hypnosis. It's no more dangerous than meditation, autogenic training, or yoga. You survive that unscathed at home too.

I've had many patients in my practice who not only handled self-hypnosis well but enjoyed it. And if a patient enjoys doing self-hypnosis, no matter how simple the suggestion may seem, it's a very good support for compliance. Discuss the process once before hypnosis and give the client a short, keyword list of the steps of self-hypnosis to take home, so they have a small guide.

+++ End of Guidelines +++

Now you're learning how to do self-hypnosis... This is very easy because you're already in trance; you're experiencing hypnosis right now... So, it's about teaching your body to reach this state very easily again... whenever you want to use self-hypnosis for yourself... and you can use it... You can use it every day... And with the help of self-hypnosis, you can set yourself more and more to calmness and serenity every day... you can let go of fearful thoughts and fearful expectations every day, even before they can arise... I'll show you how to do it, and then you can use self-hypnosis again and again... It's really easy, and you are completely safe... because now you're learning how to do it... You can decide for yourself when and where you go into a nice and liberating trance... Isn't that great?...

Now, enjoy the inner calm... This is hypnosis... You know it, and you're experiencing it right now... a truly pleasant state that you can experience at home too... for this, you use a trigger, a tool... You always have it with you; it's your right hand... Now close your right hand into a fist... [Wait until the client follows the prompt] ... Good... And now we're going to connect opening your fist with hypnosis...

Keep your hand closed... Your subconscious is now learning that the deliberate closing and opening of your right hand is the signal to immediately go into a pleasant state of trance... Whenever you make yourself comfortable to experience self-hypnosis and then close your right hand into a fist and open it with the words... I am going into trance immediately... you actually go immediately into the state of trance that feels just like now... So, now open your hand slowly and whisper... I am going into trance immediately... [Wait until the client has done that] ... Good...

Now, you deepen your self-hypnosis by whispering... I am going into trance one more time... I am going into trance two more times... I am going into trance three more times... and so on... until you finally reach ten and whisper... I am going into trance ten more times... and you sink deeper and deeper into the state of trance... A part of you goes into a truly beautiful, deep trance, and another part stays awake and guides you through the trance... Everything is completely safe and fine...

We come to the main part of self-hypnosis, the crucial part, because now you can ensure that you turn off fearful expectations... You work in this part with a suggestion that frees you... You whisper this ten times in a row... Ten times you say... I say goodbye to fear because I want to live free and relaxed... Again, you count... You say... I say goodbye to fear because I want to live free and relaxed one more time... I say goodbye to fear because I want to live free and relaxed two more times... I say goodbye to fear because I want to live free and relaxed three more times... until you whisper... I say goodbye to fear because I want to live free and relaxed ten more times... and then you feel free...

To end the self-hypnosis, imagine standing with bare feet in deep snow... Your soles are getting ice cold... Then you say loudly and clearly... Stop now, I'm waking up... and then you count loudly and clearly to three and open your eyes... It's really easy... So, once again... To end the self-hypnosis, imagine standing with bare feet in deep snow and say... Stop now, I'm waking up—One—Two—Three... and then you're awake and open your eyes... It's that simple...

You can now end those fearful thoughts yourself... You can end any fear—with self-hypnosis... Your subconscious has learned for you to go immediately into trance with a trigger, and you know what you have to do... You make yourself comfortable and close your eyes because you want to go into trance, and you close your hand into a fist... You open your hand with the words... I am going into trance immediately... and deepen the calmness with the words I am going into trance even deeper... Then follows the suggestion... I say goodbye to fear because I want to live free and relaxed... and then you imagine snow on your feet and say... Stop now, I'm waking up—One—Two—Three...

Hypnosis 10

We're constantly searching for new paths... for changes in our lives... We search externally and look around us... learn from other people or from role models... or by recognizing in others what we don't want and which paths we don't want to take... On an inner journey, we can learn differently... in the inner encounter with ourselves... In our imagination, we find a place where we can learn better and faster than in our everyday life because our feelings hold all our life experiences... Today, you can take such a journey, you can dive into your own imagination and experience this special place: the land of dreams... Imagine you're moving through space and time... through thoughts and feelings... through memories and fantasy... and you arrive in the land of dreams... at the most beautiful place you can imagine... in the middle of nature... You hear birds singing, and you hear the gentle sound of a small river in the background... The wind blows through the branches of the trees and hums a little melody... You're in the land of dreams...

You're standing on a path that winds between blooming trees... You follow this path, step by step... The trees bloom in beautiful colors... You think about the blossoms of life... about all that is new... about all the opportunities and possibilities that have been in your life and that will always be... Sometimes we pass by the blossoms of life, leaving them unnoticed... Then they wither away, and one day we encounter new opportunities and possibilities that again show themselves as blossoms... Each blossom turns into a beautiful and ripe fruit when the right time comes... and maybe today is the right time to seize an opportunity... maybe today this special chance is within reach... You think about fear... It has been with you for a long time... Often, it came unexpectedly and suddenly, surprising and overwhelming you... Then, over time, you began to fear the next panic attack... This expectation was also oppressive... this anticipation of fear, or as therapists say, this anticipatory anxiety... You walk toward a station... It's an old station that suddenly and unexpectedly appears behind the blooming trees... It's almost hidden here among the trees, but you found it... or it found you, who knows... You walk toward the station... There is only one track... and a platform... No one else is here... You walk onto the platform and look into the distance... Your gaze follows the track... You look in both directions and can see very far... But there's no train approaching... You look around and wonder why there's a station here, in the middle of blooming trees... Then you see a sign that says... Station of Fear, please wait... That's how it felt to you in the last few years/months/weeks [Please adjust to the duration of the previous anticipation of fear] ... You've waited and waited... You've repeatedly waited for fear as if it were inevitable... Inevitable, you had indeed experienced many panic attacks... Then you thought the fear would return someday, and you waited... But often, it didn't come... It never actually came when you expected it... It always came suddenly... Perhaps you thought that if you waited for it, it wouldn't be able to surprise and overwhelm you so dramatically... So, you were here... In your thoughts and in your feelings, you were here at the station of fear and did exactly what the sign said... You waited... The train of fear didn't come, and it's not coming today either... You look at the station of fear more closely, walking up and down... It looks very old, like stations used to be... And it's already worn out and slowly falling apart... It's gradually crumbling...

Now you notice that the track bed also looks like it hasn't served any purpose for a long time... Grass has long since grown through the ties and is overgrowing them... Nature is slowly reclaiming this place... That's how it feels inside you... Your nature, without anticipatory anxiety and without panic attacks, is gradually reclaiming this place of fear because it is no longer needed... You decide not to wait here any longer... You look at the sign again... It reflects your thoughts, your feelings... The sign has changed, because everything changes in the land of dreams in a single moment when the right time has come... Today is the right time... Now is the right moment... The sign now says... Station of Liberation, please move on... That's what you're doing today... You're not standing still any longer; you're moving on... You're walking back to the blooming trees... You find a tree that's even further along than the others... It's already bearing ripe fruit... an apple tree... Red apples hang on the tree... You pick a ripe red apple and take a bite... It tastes wonderfully sweet... You look up into the bright blue sky, which is vast and open... The sun is shining... You look once more at the station and hear a crunching sound... then the old station of fear with the platform of waiting crumbles to dust before your eyes... You look around and find a new path that leads you to more and more trees with ripe fruits... You see peaches and oranges... pears and cherries... Everything shines in new and vibrant colors, and you feel free... You're no longer waiting, you're moving on...

Here in the land of dreams, it's easy; here every good thought becomes reality... Here, fears and anticipatory anxiety crumble to dust if you want them to... But it's not only possible here; it's also possible in reality because the land of dreams is a reality... it's not a fairy tale, not an invention... The land of dreams is the reality within you... It's the truth of your feelings... The land of dreams lies deep within you and has always been there... always... I'm just telling you about it...

Distribution, publication, and copying in any form are prohibited and subject to damages.

All Titles in the Series

Volume 1: Smoking Cessation
Volume 2: Anxiety and Restlessness
Volume 3: Burnout
Volume 4: Reducing Overweight
Volume 5: Coping with the Past
Volume 6: Suicidal Thoughts and Attempts
Volume 7: Psycho-Oncology
Volume 8: Obsessions and Tics
Volume 9: Self-Confidence and Decision-Making
Volume 10: Grief Work
Volume 11: Psychosomatics
Volume 12: Chronic Pain
Volume 13: Depressive Thoughts
Volume 14: Panic Attacks
Volume 15: Domestic Violence, Victim Support
Volume 16: Post-Traumatic Stress
Volume 17: Exam Anxiety and Stage Fright
Volume 18: Anti-Violence Training, Offender Support
Volume 19: Addiction Tendencies
Volume 20: Social Phobia and Fear of Contact
Volume 21: Nail Biting
Volume 22: Self-Awareness and Self-Love
Volume 23: Teeth Grinding and Night Clenching
Volume 24: Feelings of Guilt
Volume 25: Fear in Crowds
Volume 26: Fear of Flying, Aviophobia
Volume 27: Fear in Enclosed Spaces, Claustrophobia
Volume 28: Tinnitus, Ear Noises
Volume 29: Fear of Heights
Volume 30: Neurodermatitis

Copying, publishing, and sharing with third parties are only permitted with the written consent of the author. Please observe the notes on copyright and usage.

Volume 31: Finding Inner Balance
Volume 32: Overcoming Loneliness
Volume 33: Fear of Illness, Hypochondria
Volume 34: Anticipatory Anxiety, Fear of Fear
Volume 35: Jealousy in Relationships
Volume 36: Driving Anxiety
Volume 37: New Start after Separation
Volume 38: Fear of Injections
Volume 39: Heart Anxiety Neurosis
Volume 40: Overcoming Resentment and Anger
Volume 41: Resolving Blockages and Positive Thinking
Volume 42: Stress Reduction, Stress Management
Volume 43: Body Relaxation
Volume 44: Deep Relaxation
Volume 45: Fear of the Dark
Volume 46: Falling Asleep and Staying Asleep
Volume 47: Compulsive Buying
Volume 48: Restless Legs Syndrome
Volume 49: Bulimia
Volume 50: Anorexia
Volume 51: Overcoming Nightmares
Volume 52: Imagined Deformity
Volume 53: Overcoming Distrust, Finding Trust
Volume 54: Processing Failures
Volume 55: Humiliation, Emotional Hurt
Volume 56: Distressing Compassion, Vicarious Suffering
Volume 57: Self-Forgiveness
Volume 58: Self-Awareness, Self-Confidence
Volume 59: Saying No
Volume 60: Assertiveness
Volume 61: Setting Boundaries and Self-Assertion
Volume 62: Decision-Making Ability

Volume 63: Success Orientation
Volume 64: Ruminating, Circular Thinking
Volume 65: Accepting Pregnancy
Volume 66: Birth Preparation
Volume 67: Spiritual Opening
Volume 68: Joy of Life and Inner Lightness
Volume 69: Patience and Inner Peace
Volume 70: Fibromyalgia and Rheumatism
Volume 71: Irritable Bowel Syndrome, Crohn's Disease
Volume 72: Fear of Nausea, Emetophobia
Volume 73: Stuttering and Cluttering, Speech Flow Disorders
Volume 74: Concentration and Knowledge Anchoring
Volume 75: Vitality and Spontaneity
Volume 76: Searching for Meaning and Finding Goals
Volume 77: Life Crises, Life Events
Volume 78: Workaholism, Goal Obsession
Volume 79: Helper Syndrome, Helpless Helpers
Volume 80: Medication Abuse
Volume 81: Gambling Addiction
Volume 82: Internet Addiction, Smartphone Addiction
Volume 83: Hoarding Disorder, Compulsive Collecting
Volume 84: Conspiracy Thoughts, Overvalued Ideas
Volume 85: Fear of Operations and Treatments
Volume 86: Fear of Aging
Volume 87: Travel Anxiety
Volume 88: Anxiety When Urinating, Paruresis
Volume 89: Fear of Intimacy and Togetherness
Volume 90: Fear of Blushing
Volume 91: Coming Out in Homosexuality
Volume 92: Charisma Training
Volume 93: Migraines and Chronic Headaches
Volume 94: Overcoming Allergies, Bronchial Asthma

Volume 95: Normalizing Blood Pressure
Volume 96: Compulsive Perfectionism
Volume 97: Sports Hypnosis, Motivation
Volume 98: Sports Hypnosis, Performance Enhancement
Volume 99: Determination and Focus
Volume 100: Encountering the Inner Child
Volume 101: Cravings, Binge Eating
Volume 102: Stimulating Metabolism
Volume 103: Bipolar Mood Swings
Volume 104: Borderline, Identity Crises
Volume 105: Hypomania, Euphoria, Mania
Volume 106: Restlessness, Agitation
Volume 107: Nervous Breakdown
Volume 108: Adjustment Disorders
Volume 109: Self-Alienation, Depersonalization
Volume 110: Ending Self-Pity
Volume 111: Primary Gain of Illness
Volume 112: Secondary Gain of Illness
Volume 113: Bullying, Victim Support
Volume 114: Letting Go of Envy and Jealousy
Volume 115: Fear of Spiders, Arachnophobia
Volume 116: Fear of Dogs or Cats
Volume 117: Fear of Strangers, Xenophobia
Volume 118: Excessive Worries, Generalized Anxiety
Volume 119: Strengthening Sense of Responsibility
Volume 120: Unrequited Love, Heartache
Volume 121: Work-Life Balance
Volume 122: Letting Go of Unattainable Goals
Volume 123: Allowing and Accepting Help
Volume 124: Letting Go of Adult Children
Volume 125: Tourette Syndrome
Volume 126: Life Changes and New Starts

Volume 127: Accepting Life in a Wheelchair
Volume 128: Understanding and Overcoming Homesickness
Volume 129: Understanding and Overcoming Wanderlust
Volume 130: Dizziness, Meniere's Disease
Volume 131: Overcoming Aggression
Volume 132: Cutting and Self-Harm
Volume 133: Hair Pulling, Trichotillomania
Volume 134: Postpartum Depression
Volume 135: For Relatives of Dementia Patients
Volume 136: Self-Harm, Artificial Disorders
Volume 137: Activating Self-Healing Powers
Volume 138: Preventing Depression Relapse
Volume 139: Reactive Psychoses, Follow-Up
Volume 140: Obsessive Thoughts and Impulses
Volume 141: Compulsive Checking
Volume 142: Compulsive Counting, Symmetry Obsession
Volume 143: Compulsive Washing, Cleanliness Obsession
Volume 144: Compulsive Questioning
Volume 145: Dissociative Paralysis
Volume 146: Phantom Pain
Volume 147: Overcoming Complaining
Volume 148: Hay Fever, Pollen Allergy
Volume 149: Sexual Abuse, Victim Support
Volume 150: Standing Strong Against Sexism, #metoo
Volume 151: Binge Eating
Volume 152: Overcoming Thoughts of Revenge
Volume 153: Detachment from the Aggressor, Stockholm Syndrome
Volume 154: Courage to Separate
Volume 155: Chronic Fatigue, Exhaustion
Volume 156: Fear of the Future, Existential Anxiety
Volume 157: Excessive Worry About Children
Volume 158: Fear of Failure

Volume 159: Ending Distrust and Control
Volume 160: Dejection, Dysphoria
Volume 161: Boreout, Chronic Boredom
Volume 162: Bipolar Disorders, Relapse Prevention
Volume 163: Mania, Relapse Prevention
Volume 164: Nihilism, Feelings of Worthlessness
Volume 165: Thumb Sucking
Volume 166: Being Brave
Volume 167: Being Proud
Volume 168: Overcoming Shyness
Volume 169: Being Able to Delegate Responsibility
Volume 170: Being Able to Show Emotions
Volume 171: Letting Go of Guilt, Victim Support
Volume 172: Processing Guilt, Offender Support
Volume 173: Mood Swings, Cyclothymia
Volume 174: Lack of Drive, Vital Sadness
Volume 175: Hearing Voices with Reality Reference
Volume 176: Confident Communication
Volume 177: Standing Up for Oneself
Volume 178: Taking New Paths
Volume 179: Confident Job Application
Volume 180: No Longer Being Taken Advantage Of
Volume 181: End of Submissiveness
Volume 182: Depressive Numbness
Volume 183: Mood Drops, Affective Incontinence
Volume 184: Mood Instability
Volume 185: Somatoform Disorders
Volume 186: Stomach Ulcer, Psychosomatic
Volume 187: Accepting Amputation
Volume 188: Overcoming and Letting Go of Hatred
Volume 189: Ending Accusations
Volume 190: Allowing Tears, Being Able to Cry

Volume 191: Finding and Sorting Repressed Feelings
Volume 192: Somatoform Pain
Volume 193: Living Autonomously
Volume 194: Anhedonia, Joylessness
Volume 195: Persistent Sadness
Volume 196: Obesity, Food Addiction
Volume 197: Parents of Abused Children
Volume 198: Letting Go and Letting Be
Volume 199: Childhood Sexual Abuse
Volume 200: Fear of Loss

www.ingramcontent.com/pod-product-compliance
Lightning Source LLC
Chambersburg PA
CBHW030503220526
45464CB00006B/2630